The Canadian Red C

Basic Life Support
The ABC's of First Aid

SUDDENLY SAFE SERVICES
FIRST AID & CPR TRAINING
Siegrid Goodrich
941-2506

ul 880 3709

The Canadian Red Cross Society

Basic Life Support

The ABC's of First Aid

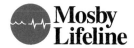

St. Louis Baltimore Boston Chicago London Madrid Philadelphia Sydney Toronto

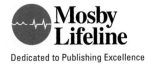

Mosby Lifeline

Dedicated to Publishing Excellence

Printed in the United States of America

Composition by Clarinda Company
Colour separation by Color Dot Graphics, Inc.
Printing/binding by William C. Brown

Mosby–Year Book, Inc.
11830 Westline Industrial Drive
St. Louis, Missouri 63146

International Standard Book Number 0-8016-7951-6

93 94 95 96 97 98 / 9 8 7 6 5 4 3 2 1

Acknowledgements

The Canadian Red Cross Society wishes to express our appreciation to the volunteers and staff of the American National Red Cross Health and Safety Department that made this project possible. The Society also wishes to acknowledge the efforts of the many volunteers and staff involved in the Canadian development of this manual. Their commitment to excellence made this manual possible.

Revision was supplied by:
   Brian Weitzman, M.D.C.M., F.R.C.P. (C.), C.C.F.P. (E.M.)
   S. H. Knox, M.D.C.M.

Special thanks go to Tom Lochhaas, Ed.D., Developmental Editor.
External review and guidance was provided by the following individuals:
   Merle Blizzard, R.N., Canadian Red Cross Society Instructor Trainer
   Barney Chandra, Canadian Red Cross Society Instructor Trainer

The Mosby – Year Book production team included: David T. Culverwell, Publisher; Claire Merrick, Executive Editor; Christi Mangold, Developmental Editor; Gayle May Morris, Project Manager; Donna Walls, Senior Production Editor; Kay Michael Kramer, Art and Design Director; and Susan Lane, Senior Designer. Special thanks go to Steve O'Hearn, Allan Orr, and John Hirst of Times Mirror Professional Publishing.

Contents

Introduction, 1

Recognizing Emergencies, 1

Decide to Act, 1

The Emergency Medical Services System (EMS), 2

Giving First Aid, 3

Recovery Position, 5

Airway Emergencies, 6

PRACTISE SESSIONS

    First Aid for a Conscious Adult or Child with a Complete Airway Obstruction, 9

    First Aid for a Conscious Infant with a Complete Airway Obstruction, 11

    First Aid for an Unconscious Adult or Child with a Complete Airway Obstruction, 15

    First Aid for an Unconscious Infant with a Complete Airway Obstruction, 19

Breathing Emergencies, 24

PRACTISE SESSIONS

    Rescue Breathing for an Adult, 26

    Rescue Breathing for a Child, 30

    Rescue Breathing for an Infant, 34

Cardiovascular Emergencies, 38

PRACTISE SESSIONS

    CPR for an Adult, 44

    Two-Rescuer CPR for an Adult, 49

    CPR for a Child, 52

    CPR for an Infant, 56

APPENDIXES

A   Common Questions about Cardiovascular Health and First Aid, 60

B   Prevention of Injuries to Children, 62

Introduction

This booklet reviews basic first aid for airway, breathing, and cardiovascular emergencies. You may be the only person at the emergency scene who can help — you must get involved. Do not worry that you're not an expert — you can always help. Every year countless bystanders give help in emergencies. Some phone for help, some comfort the casualty or family members, some give first aid, and still others help keep order at the emergency scene. There are many things that you can do to help.

Your involvement can make the difference between life and death or between complete recovery and permanent disability. The four steps involved in giving help are:

1. Recognize that an emergency exists.
2. Decide to act.
3. Call EMS.
4. Give first aid until help arrives.

Recognizing Emergencies

An emergency can be a sudden illness that requires immediate medical attention, such as a heart attack or a serious injury. You may encounter an emergency at any time, in any place. In some cases it may be obvious; in others you may not know right away that the person is experiencing an emergency. For example, a person having a heart attack may comment that he or she is having "indigestion;" but you may recognize the signs and symptoms of a heart attack and know that the person could need emergency care.

Decide to Act

Sometimes in an emergency people hesitate to act. There are five common reasons people give for not acting. If you think about these reasons now and are mentally prepared, you will find that they may be easily overcome.

1. *Do not be discouraged by the presence of other people.* Other people at the emergency scene can cause confusion or make you think that someone else is taking care of the situation. Do not assume that someone is giving first aid, and do not feel embarrassed in front of strangers. It is much more important to help and possibly save a life.

2. *Do not let uncertainty about the casualty affect your help.* The person needing your help may be a stranger, much older or much younger than you, or of a different gender or race. The person still needs your help — do not let such concerns slow you down.

3. *Do not be discouraged by the nature of the injury or illness.* An injury or illness may be unpleasant because of blood, vomit, or torn or burned skin. If necessary, turn away for a moment and take a few deep breaths. Remember this situation is an emergency. Your help can save a life. Try to do for the casualty what you would want someone to do for you.

4. *Do not be afraid to help because you fear you may catch some disease from the casualty.* The risk of this is actually very small, and you can make the risk even smaller by protecting yourself. Avoid direct contact with a casualty's body fluids. Wash thoroughly after giving care. If you have an open wound, see your doctor if you contact a casualty's body fluids. If possible, wear disposable gloves when giving first aid.

5. *Do not hesitate out of fear that you will do something wrong or be sued.* In an emergency, you may fear that you

might do something to make the situation worse. If you call EMS and do the best that you can according to your training, you do not need to be concerned about legal problems when giving first aid. As long as you act reasonably and prudently when you give first aid, you need not worry about being sued. Most of the provinces even have laws to protect you when you act in good faith to give emergency assistance to a casualty. To do your best, follow your training in the care you give. Do not move a casualty unless the person's life is endangered, and do not abandon the casualty once you have begun to give care.

The Emergency Medical Services System (EMS)

The EMS is a coordinated system that exists throughout the country to get emergency assistance to casualties with injuries or sudden illness and to transport them to a hospital. Once you recognize the emergency, calling EMS is the most important action you and other bystanders can take. Early arrival of EMS personnel increases the casualty's chances of surviving a life-threatening emergency.

When you call EMS on 9-1-1 or your local emergency number, your call is answered by a *dispatcher*, who sends an ambulance to the scene with EMS professionals. Police, fire-fighters, and Emergency Medical Attendants (EMAs) may be dispatched to the scene. The EMA can give more advanced first aid and may use life-support techniques. *Paramedics* are highly specialized EMAs who can also give medications and intravenous fluids, give advanced airway care, and assess abnormal heart rhythms.

The EMS system varies somewhat from community to community. Although the level of training of the ambulance attendants and EMAs may vary somewhat, the principles of calling EMS are the same in all provinces.

When to Call EMS

When you have determined that there is an emergency and when you are sure the scene is safe, you must quickly check the injured or ill person to see if he or she is unresponsive. If so, the next step is to call EMS immediately before giving care. If the casualty is an infant or child, provide emergency care for up to 1 minute before calling EMS. Even if the casualty is conscious, call EMS if serious injury or illness is suspected. As a rule, call EMS personnel for any of the following conditions:

- Unconsciousness or altered level of consciousness
- Breathing problems (difficulty breathing or no breathing)
- Persistent chest pain or pressure
- No pulse
- Severe bleeding
- Vomiting blood or passing blood
- Poisoning
- Convulsions, severe headache, or slurred speech
- Injuries to head, neck, or back
- Possible broken bones

How to Call EMS

Sending someone else to call the emergency number is better because it enables you to stay with the casualty and keep giving first aid.

The local emergency number will be answered by the dispatcher in a communications center. This person quickly decides which professionals to send to the scene and may give the caller instructions on what first aid to give until help arrives. Therefore, when you tell someone to call for help, do the following:

1. Send a bystander, or possibly two, to make the call.

2. Give the caller(s) the EMS telephone number to call. This number is 9-1-1 in many places. Tell the caller(s) to dial O for the Operator only if you or the caller do not know the local emergency number. Sometimes the emergency number is on the inside front cover of the telephone book or displayed on the pay phone.

3. Tell the caller(s) what to tell the dispatcher. For example, "I have an unconscious adult here." The dispatcher will ask many questions, including the following:

   a. Where the emergency is located. Give the exact address or location, the names of nearby intersecting streets, landmarks, the name of the building, the floor, the room number, and any other information needed to ensure that EMS personnel can find you.

   b. Telephone number from which the call is being made and any other available phone number for a call back.

   c. Caller's name.

   d. What has happened.

   e. How many people are involved.

   f. Condition of the casualty — for example, chest pain, trouble breathing, no pulse. The dispatcher will ask if the person is conscious and breathing and the person's approximate age.

   g. The first aid being given.

4. Tell the caller(s) not to hang up until the dispatcher hangs up.

5. Tell the caller(s) to report to you after making the call and tell you what the dispatcher said.

If you are alone with the casualty, call out loudly for help to attract someone who can help by making this call. If no one comes, get to a phone as fast as you can to call EMS. Then return to the casualty to keep giving help. With an infant or child under the age of 8, give emergency care for up to 1 minute first, and then go to the telephone to call EMS. Take the infant or child with you to the telephone.

Emergency Cardiac Care

Heart attacks are one of the most common and most serious medical emergencies for the EMS system. Each year 50,000 Canadians die of heart attacks; one half of these deaths occur before the casualty reaches the hospital. With your training, one of the most important things you can do is be prepared to give emergency cardiac care. This consists of:

- Recognizing the signs and symptoms of heart attack
- Promptly calling EMS
- Starting basic life support immediately (including CPR if needed)
- Early difibrillation (if needed)
- EMAs giving advanced cardiac life support as soon as possible
- Transporting the casualty to the hospital by ambulance

The key to survival for such a casualty is quick activation of the EMS system.

Giving First Aid

In any non trauma emergency follow four basic emergency action principles.

1. Survey the Scene.

Once you recognize an emergency, make sure the scene is safe. Look for anything that may threaten your safety and the safety of others, such as downed power lines, falling

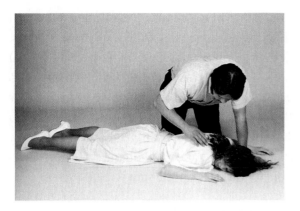

Figure 1 Determine if the person is conscious by gently tapping and asking, "Are you okay?"

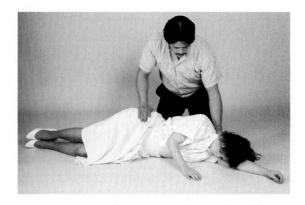

Figure 2 If the casualty's position keeps you from checking the ABCs, roll the casualty gently onto the back while supporting the head and neck.

rocks, traffic, fire, smoke, dangerous fumes, extreme weather, and deep or fast water. *If any kind of danger is threatening, do not approach the casualty. Call EMS immediately for professional help.*

Do not move a casualty unless he or she is in immediate danger, such as from fire or poisonous fumes. If you must move the casualty, do so as quickly as possible.

2. Check the Casualty for Unresponsiveness.

Start by determining if the casualty is conscious. Gently tap the person and ask, "Are you okay?" (Figure 1). Do not jostle or move the casualty. A casualty who does not respond may be unconscious; unconsciousness may indicate a life-threatening condition.

3. If the Person Does Not Respond, Call EMS.

Call 9-1-1 or your local emergency number for EMS. If possible, send someone else to call while you give care to the casualty.

4. Check the Casualty's Airway, Breathing, and Circulation (ABCs).

In any emergency you must check for airway, breathing, or circulation emergencies (the ABCs). Try to check the ABCs without moving the casualty. Only if necessary, should you roll the casualty gently onto his or her back, keeping the head and spine in as straight a line as possible (Figure 2).

A—Check the airway

Be sure the casualty has an open airway. Any person who can speak or cry is conscious and has an open airway. If the person is unconscious, ensure the airway is open by using the head-tilt/chin-lift (see Figure 7 on p. 14). This moves the tongue away from the back of the throat and lets air reach the lungs. If head or neck trauma is suspected, use the jaw thrust to open the airway. When the person's airway is blocked by food or some object, remove the blockage first.

B—Check breathing

Someone who can speak or cry is breathing. Watch an unconscious person carefully.

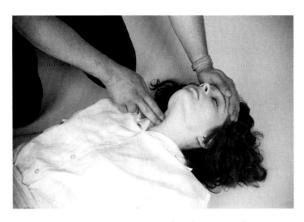

Figure 3 Determine if the heart is beating by feeling for a carotid pulse on the side of the neck closest to you.

Look to see if the chest is rising and falling, and *listen* and *feel* for breathing. Place your face close so you can hear and feel air coming out the nose and mouth. Take 3 to 5 seconds to do this. If the casualty is not breathing, you must use rescue breathing to help the person to breathe.

C—Check circulation

If the casualty is breathing, the heart is beating and you do not need to check the pulse. If the person is not breathing, you must check the pulse. Feel for the pulse in the **carotid artery** in the neck on the side closest to you (Figure 3). To find the pulse, find the Adam's apple and slide your fingers into the groove at the side of the neck. The pulse may be hard to find if it is slow or weak. If at first you do not find a pulse, start again at the Adam's apple and slide your fingers into place. When you think you are in the right spot, keep feeling for at least 5 to 10 seconds.

For infants you should check the brachial pulse inside the upper arm, not the carotid pulse in the neck. Place two fingers close to

the bone on the underside of the arm, nearer the armpit than the elbow. Press gently and feel for the pulse for 5 to 10 seconds. It is very difficult to find a pulse in infants under the age of 1 year. Therefore, unless you have special training, you should not spend more than a few seconds searching for a pulse in an infant who has stopped breathing.

If the casualty does not have a pulse, you must begin chest compressions (see p. 46).

Recovery Position

The recovery position, also called the *drainage position*, is used for unconscious casualties (1) who have an open airway, (2) who are breathing, (3) who have a pulse, and (4) who are not thought to have a neck or back injury. These casualties are positioned on their side to keep the airway open and to allow drainage from the mouth if the casualty vomits or is bleeding. Use the recovery position for these casualties even if you first used the chin lift or jaw thrust to open the airway, because in this position the airway will stay open without you having to hold the chin in position.

Follow these steps to move the unconscious casualty into the recovery position from a position on the back:
1. Raise the arm closest to you over the casualty's head.
2. Raise the knee of the leg further away from you.
3. Support the head and neck with one hand as you pull the person toward you with your other hand on the raised knee (Fig. 4, *A*).
4. Position the casualty on his or her side with knee out in front and hip at right angle to prevent the person from rolling onto his or her face (Figure 4, *B*).

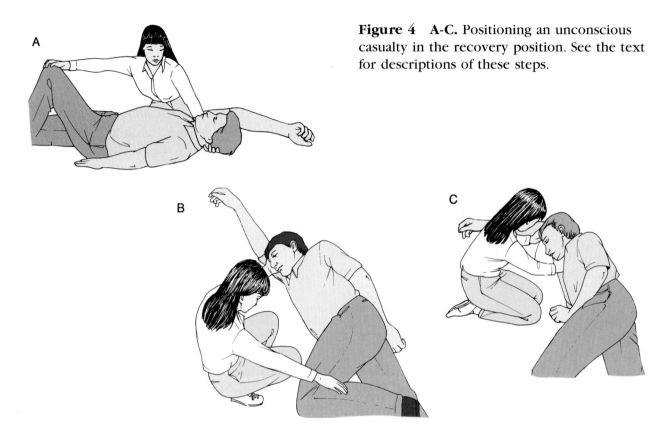

Figure 4 A-C. Positioning an unconscious casualty in the recovery position. See the text for descriptions of these steps.

5. Move the casualty's other arm into a position of comfort in front of the body.
6. With the casualty's head resting on the extended arm, tilt the head and open mouth to clear the way for drainage (Figure 4, *C*).

Airway Emergencies

If the airway is obstructed, there is no air reaching the lungs. An obstructed airway is a life-threatening emergency that requires immediate care.

Anatomy and Physiology of the Airway

Figure 5 shows how the air passes from the nose and mouth to the lungs. Air moves through the trachea (windpipe) to the bron-chi, which branch into smaller passages in the lungs.

Causes of Airway Obstruction

The most common cause of an airway obstruction in an unconscious person is the tongue, which has dropped to the back of the throat and blocked the airway. The airway can also be blocked by a foreign object, such as a piece of food, a small toy, or fluids like vomit, blood, mucus, or saliva. This is called *choking*. An airway obstruction can also occur if swollen tissues of the mouth and throat block the airway. This may occur after an injury or as the result of a severe allergic reaction.

Common causes of choking include:
• Trying to swallow large pieces of food without chewing them adequately

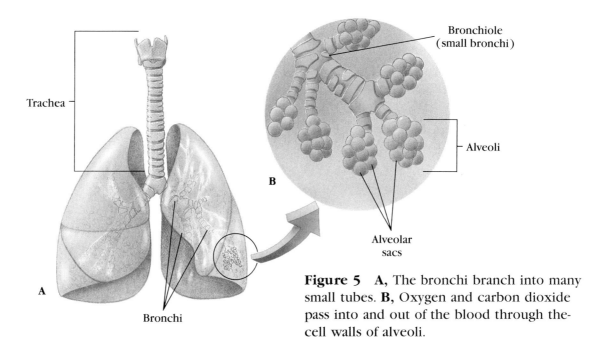

Trachea

B

Bronchiole (small bronchi)

Alveoli

Alveolar sacs

A

Bronchi

Figure 5 A, The bronchi branch into many small tubes. **B,** Oxygen and carbon dioxide pass into and out of the blood through the cell walls of alveoli.

- Drinking alcohol in excess before or during meals, making choking on food more likely
- Wearing dentures, which makes it difficult to sense whether food is fully chewed
- Eating while talking excitedly or laughing, or eating too quickly
- Walking, playing, or running with food or objects in the mouth

PREVENTION

Choking

Choking can usually be prevented by following these guidelines:
- Chew food well before swallowing, and eat slowly and calmly. Be especially careful if you have dentures. Avoid talking or laughing with food in your mouth.
- Minimize alcohol consumption before and during meals.

- Avoid walking and other physical activities with food in your mouth.
- Keep small objects out of reach of little children.

Infants and young children are particularly at risk for choking. See the guidelines in Appendix B for prevention.

Signs and Symptoms of Choking

A person with a partial airway obstruction can often get enough air into the lungs to try to dislodge the object by coughing. The person may also be able to speak. The following are signs and symptoms of a partial obstruction:
- High-pitched or wheezing sounds (stridor) when trying to breathe in
- Coughing
- Clutching at the throat with one or both hands in the universal distress signal for choking

A casualty with a complete airway obstruction has these signs and symptoms:

- Unable to breathe
- Unable to speak
- Unable to cough
- Face may appear bluish
- May be conscious or unconscious

A conscious adult can usually indicate that he or she is choking. With an infant or small child who is conscious but suddenly not able to breathe, assume the child is choking.

FIRST AID
Conscious Choking Casualty

For a casualty with a partial airway obstruction, do not interfere with attempts to cough up the object. A person who can cough or speak is getting enough air to breathe. Encourage continued coughing. If coughing persists, call EMS. If the person is barely able to breathe, the cough is very weak, and he or she cannot speak at all, treat this as a complete airway obstruction.

If the casualty is choking on a foreign object, you must open the airway as quickly as possible. Use abdominal thrusts to force air from the lungs to push the object out, like a cork from a bottle of champagne (Figure 6). The method you use depends on whether the casualty is conscious or unconscious and is an adult, child, or infant. See Appendix A for variations for large adults and pregnant women.

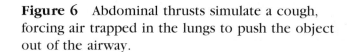

Figure 6 Abdominal thrusts simulate a cough, forcing air trapped in the lungs to push the object out of the airway.

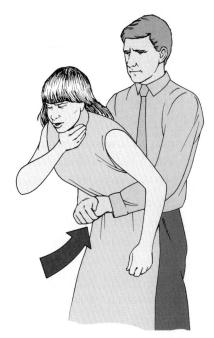

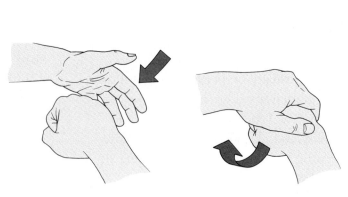

First Aid for a Conscious Adult or Child with a Complete Airway Obstruction

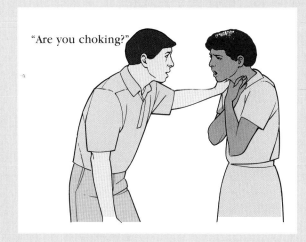

☐ **Determine if the person is choking**

- Ask, "Are you choking?"

If person is not choking . . .
- **Encourage person to continue coughing.**
- **Continue to monitor situation.**

If person is choking . . .

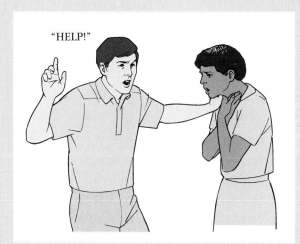

☐ **Shout for help**

- Summon someone who can help and call EMS for you as necessary.

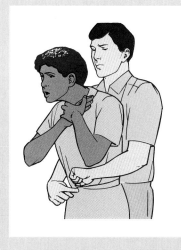

☐ **Give abdominal thrusts**

- Wrap your arms around person's waist.
- Make a fist.
- Place thumb side of fist against middle of person's abdomen just above navel and well below lower tip of breastbone.
- Grasp fist with your other hand.
- Pull fist into person's abdomen with a quick upward thrust.
- Each thrust should be a separate and distinct attempt to dislodge object.

Repeat abdominal thrusts until . . .
- Object is coughed up.
- Person starts to breathe or cough forcefully.
- Person becomes unconscious.
- EMS or other trained person takes over.

When person becomes unconscious . . .
- Shout for help.
- Summon someone who can help and ask them to call EMS.
- If alone, make the call yourself.
- If you have a child casualty, continue care for 1 minute, then make the call yourself.
- Follow these steps as clearly illustrated on page 17.
  - Do a finger sweep.
  - Attempt to ventilate, if unsuccessful . . .
  - Reopen airway and try again.
  - If air still does not go in . . .
  - Deliver up to 5 abdominal thrusts.
- Repeat these three steps until successful.

First Aid for a Conscious Infant with a Complete Airway Obstruction

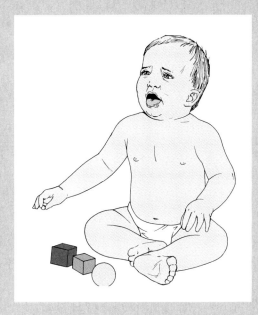

☐ **Determine if the infant is choking**

- Observe if the infant cannot breathe, cough, or cry, or is coughing weakly or making high-pitched sounds.

If infant is not choking . . .
- **Let the infant keep coughing.**
- **Continue to monitor situation.**

If infant is choking . . .

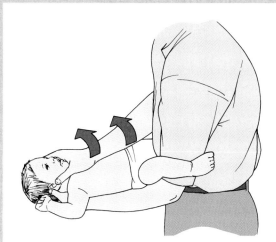

☐ **Turn infant face down**

- Support infant's head and neck.
- Turn infant face down on your forearm with head lower than the body.

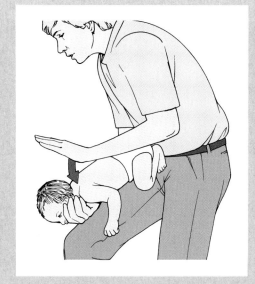

☐ **Give 5 back blows**

- Lower your forearm onto your thigh.
- Give 5 back blows forcefully between infant's shoulder blades with the heel of your hand.

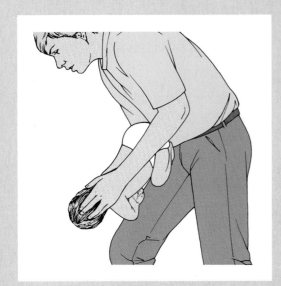

☐ Turn infant onto back

- Support back of infant's head and neck.
- Turn infant onto back in your lap with head supported lower than body.

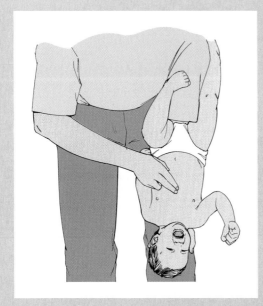

☐ Give 5 chest thrusts

- Find correct finger position.
- Place middle three fingers with index finger on the line between the nipples.
- Lift index finger, so that the middle and ring fingers are on sternum below the nipple line.
- Quickly compress breastbone 1.3 to 2.5 cm (0.5 to 1 inch) for 5 thrusts.

Repeat back blows and chest thrusts until . . .
- Object is coughed up.
- Infant starts to cry, breathe, or cough forcefully.
- Infant becomes unconscious
- EMS or other trained person takes over.

When infant becomes unconscious . . .
- Shout for help.
- Summon someone who can help and call EMS.
- If alone, continue care for 1 minute, then call EMS.
- Follow these steps as clearly illustrated on pp. 21 and 22.
  ◦ Do a finger sweep.
  ◦ Attempt to ventilate, if unsuccesful . . .
  ◦ Reopen airway and try again.
  ◦ If air still does not go in . . .
  ◦ Deliver 5 back blows and 5 chest thrusts.
- Repeat these 3 steps until successful.

First Aid for Unconscious Choking Casualty

If the casualty is unconscious or becomes unconscious while you are giving care, first aid includes opening the airway.

Opening the airway: head-tilt/chin-lift

If the casualty is unconscious and the airway is blocked by the tongue, open the airway by tilting the head back and lifting the chin; this is the head-tilt/chin-lift method. If the airway is blocked by swollen tissues, you may not be able to open the airway. Arriving EMS professionals will care for this problem.

The head-tilt/chin-lift method positions the throat so that the tongue does not block the airway. If the casualty may have other injuries, check for breathing before moving the person to avoid causing further harm. Then, if the casualty is not breathing, support the head and neck with one hand while rolling the person onto the back with the other. With the person lying flat on the back, tilt the head back with one hand on the casualty's forehead and raise the chin

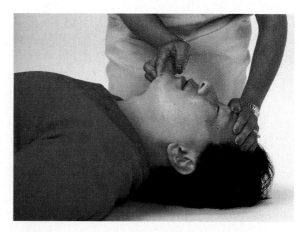

Figure 7   The head-tilt/chin-lift method is used for opening the airway.

with your other hand (Figure 7). Pinch the nostrils closed, seal your mouth over the casualty's, and give two breaths (see p. 16). If the breaths go in, the person does not have an obstructed airway. If breaths do not go in, retilt the person's head and repeat the breaths. If the breaths still do not go in, the person has an airway obstruction and needs first aid for choking.

First Aid for an Unconscious Adult or Child with a Complete Airway Obstruction

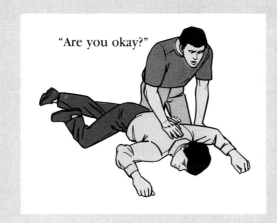

☐ Check for responsiveness

- Tap or gently shake person.
- Shout, "Are you OK?"

If person does not respond . . .

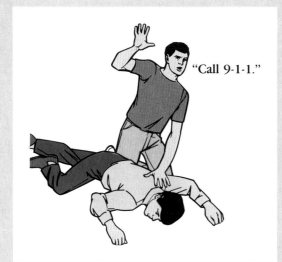

☐ Shout for help and call EMS

- Summon someone who can help and call EMS or call EMS yourself.
- With a child, continue care for 1 minute and then call EMS.

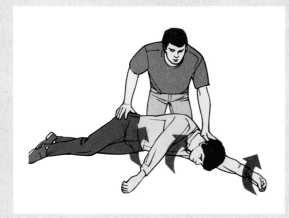

☐ Roll person onto back (if necessary)

- Kneel facing person.
- Use one hand to cradle the head and neck, and place the other hand on the person's hip.
- Roll person toward you, moving as a single unit. Remember to support the back of head and neck.

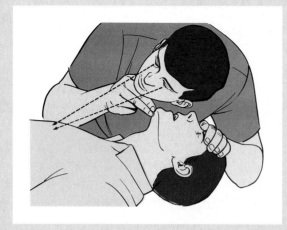

☐ Open airway and check for breathing

- Tilt head back and lift chin.
- Look, listen, and feel for breathing for 3 to 5 seconds.

If person is breathing . . .
- **Put the casualty in the recovery position.**
- **Keep airway open.**
- **Monitor breathing.**

If person is not breathing . . .

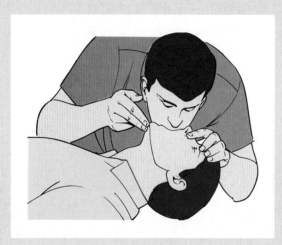

☐ Give 2 slow breaths

- Pinch nose shut and seal your lips tightly around person's mouth.
- Give 2 slow breaths, allowing 1 1/2 to 2 seconds per breath.
- Watch chest rise to see that your breaths go in.

If breaths go in . . .
- **Check pulse.**
- **If person has a pulse but is not breathing, do rescue breathing.**
- **If person has no pulse and is not breathing, do CPR.**

If breaths do not go in . . .

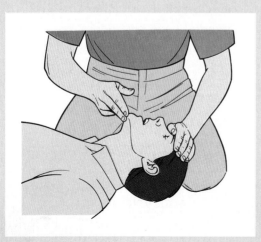

☐ Retilt person's head and repeat breaths

- Tilt person's head farther back.
- Pinch nose shut and seal your lips tightly around person's mouth.
- Give 2 slow breaths.

If breaths still do not go in . . .

☐ Give 5 abdominal thrusts

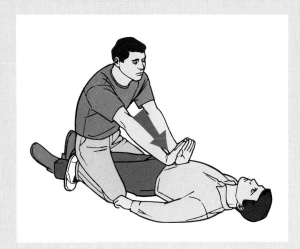

- Place heel of one hand just above the navel.
- Place other hand directly on top of first hand.
- Press into person's abdomen with upward thrusts.

☐ Do finger sweep

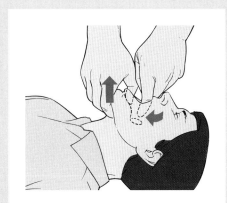

- Grasp both tongue and lower jaw between your thumb and fingers and lift jaw.
- Slide finger down inside of cheek to base of tongue.
- Attempt to sweep out object.

☐ Open airway and give 2 slow breaths

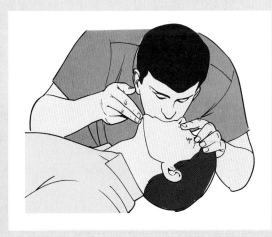

- Tilt head back.
- Pinch nose shut.
- Seal your lips tightly around person's mouth.
- Give 2 slow breaths.
- Watch chest rise to see if your breaths go in.

If breaths go in . . .
- Check pulse.
- If person has a pulse but is not breathing, do rescue breathing.
- If person has no pulse and is not breathing, do CPR.

If breaths do not go in . . .
- Repeat thrusts, finger sweep, and breathing steps until . . .
- Obstruction is removed.
- Person starts to breathe or cough.
- EMS personnel take over.

First Aid for an Unconscious Infant with a Complete Airway Obstruction

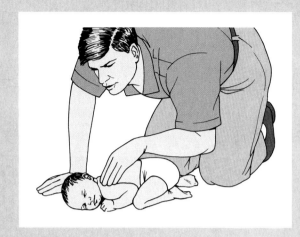

☐ Check for consciousness

- Tap the infant and call his or her name.

If the infant does not cry or otherwise respond . . .

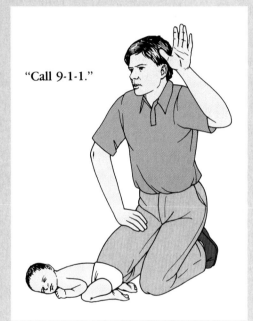

"Call 9-1-1."

☐ Shout for help

- Summon someone who can call EMS and describe infant's condition. If alone, give care for 1 minute, and then call EMS.

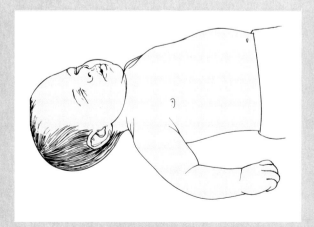

☐ Put the infant on his or her back on a firm, flat surface

19

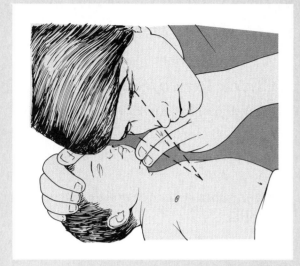

☐ Open airway and check for breathing

- Tilt head gently to "sniffing" position and lift chin.
- Look, listen, and feel for breathing for 3 to 5 seconds.

If the infant is breathing . . .
- **Position the infant in the recovery position.**
- **Keep airway open.**
- **Monitor breathing.**
- **If alone, take the infant with you to the telephone.**
- **Phone EMS and await their arrival.**

If the infant is not breathing . . .

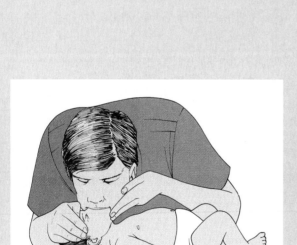

☐ Give 2 slow puffs

- Keep head tilted.
- Seal your lips tightly around the infant's nose and mouth.
- Give 2 slow puffs, allowing 1 to 1 1/2 seconds per breath.
- Watch chest rise to see that your puffs go in.

If puffs go in . . .
- **Check for pulse. If no pulse, begin CPR.**

If puffs do not go in . . .

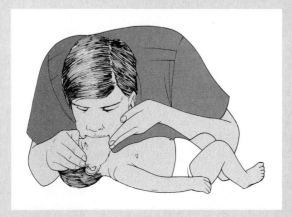

☐ Retilt infant's head and repeat puffs

- Tilt infant's head back again.
- Seal your lips tightly around the nose and mouth.
- Give 2 slow puffs.

If puffs still do not go in . . .

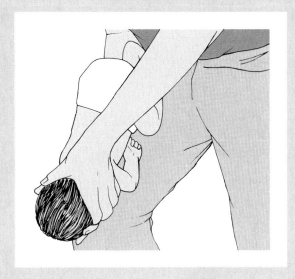

☐ Turn infant facedown

- Support infant's head and neck.
- Turn infant facedown on your forearm, head supported lower than body.

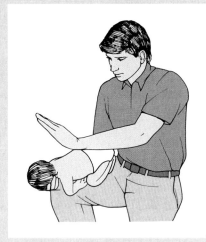

☐ Give 5 back blows

- Give 5 back blows forcefully between infant's shoulder blades with heel of hand.

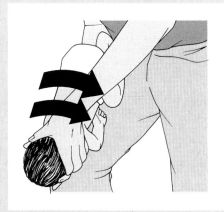

☐ Turn infant onto back

- Support back of infant's head and neck.
- Turn infant onto back in your lap with head supported lower than the body.

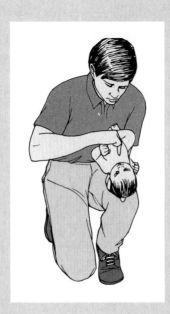

☐ Give 5 chest thrusts

- Find correct finger position.
- Place middle three fingers with index finger on the line between the nipples.
- Lift index finger, so that the middle and ring fingers are on sternum below the nipple line.
- Quickly compress the breastbone 1.3 to 2.5 cm (0.5 to 1 inch) for 5 thrusts.

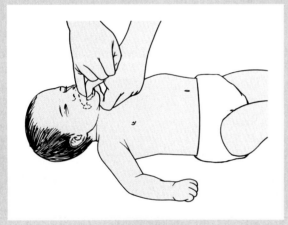

☐ Look for object in infant's throat

- Grasp the tongue and lower jaw between your thumb and fingers, and lift jaw.
- If you see an object in the throat, try to remove it with a finger sweep.

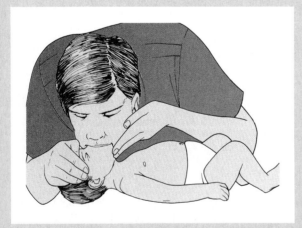

☐ Open airway and give 2 slow puffs

- Tilt head back gently to "sniffing" position and lift chin.
- Seal your lips tightly over the infant's nose and mouth.
- Give 2 slow puffs, allowing 1 to 1 1/2 seconds per breath.
- Watch chest rise to see if your puffs go in.

If puffs go in . . .
- Check pulse.
- If infant has no pulse, begin CPR.
- Phone EMS personnel for ambulance and await their arrival.

If puffs do not go in . . .
- Repeat back blows, chest thrusts, and breathing steps until . . .
- Obstruction is removed.
- Infant starts to breathe or cough.
- EMS personnel take over.

Breathing Emergencies

Breathing requires the respiratory, circulatory, nervous, and musculoskeletal systems to work together. Injuries or illnesses that affect any of these systems may impair breathing.

Anatomy and Physiology of Breathing

The body requires a constant supply of oxygen for survival. When you breathe air into your lungs, the oxygen in the air is transferred to the blood. The blood then takes the oxygen to the brain, organs, muscles, and all parts of the body. The body needs oxygen to perform its many functions. Some functions require more energy and therefore more oxygen. For example, a person with a breathing problem may have just enough energy for sitting in a chair but not enough for climbing a flight of stairs.

In *respiratory arrest*, the body receives no oxygen. After a few minutes without oxygen, body systems begin to fail. A person loses consciousness within a minute and eventually the heart muscle stops.

Causes of Breathing Emergencies

Respiratory arrest may be caused by any of the following:
• An obstructed airway (choking)
• Illness (such as pneumonia)
• Respiratory conditions (such as emphysema or asthma)
• Electrocution
• Strangulation
• Suffocation
• Shock
• Drowning
• Heart attack or heart disease
• Injury to the head, chest, or lungs
• Severe allergic reaction to food or an insect sting
• Drugs and alcohol
• Poisoning, such as inhaling or ingesting toxic substances

PREVENTION
Breathing Emergencies

Breathing emergencies can result from many different causes. Everyone should follow general safety practices to prevent injuries.
• People with asthma should always have their medication with them or nearby in case of an attack. Parents of asthmatic children should take all necessary steps to ensure that others who supervise their children know about the asthma and how to assist with medications.
• People who know they have severe allergies should be careful to avoid the substances or foods that cause the allergic reaction. If they have a severe allergy to insect bites and stings, they should carry their medication with them and wear a Medic-Alert bracelet.
• Chest injuries and other injuries that lead to respiratory arrest can often be prevented by good safety practices in all areas of life, including driving motor vehicles, sports and recreational activities, working around the home, and occupational activities.
• See Appendix B for precautions to take to prevent breathing emergencies in infants and small children.
• Always seek treatment before an illness becomes an emergency. Get regular checkups and always follow the doctor's advice for use of medications.

Signs and Symptoms of Respiratory Arrest

- Unconsciousness
- Bluish appearance of the face
- Absence of chest and abdominal movement
- Absence of breath sounds

FIRST AID
Respiratory Arrest

Rescue breathing is given to casualties who are not breathing but still have a pulse. Rescue breathing works because the air you breathe into the casualty has enough oxygen to keep the person alive. The air you breath in has 21% oxygen. The air you breathe out has about 16% oxygen, which is more than enough to keep someone alive. Rescue breathing techniques are similar for an adult, child, or infant with slight variations.

Rescue Breathing for an Adult

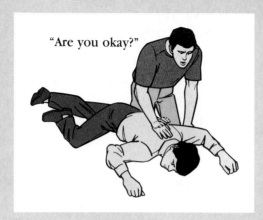

☐ **Check for unresponsiveness**
- Tap or gently shake person.
- Shout, "Are you OK?"

If person does not respond . . .

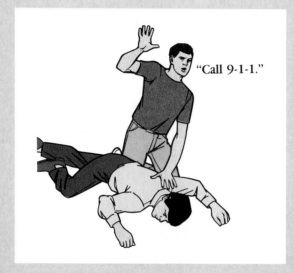

☐ **Shout for help and call EMS**
- Summon someone who can help and call EMS.

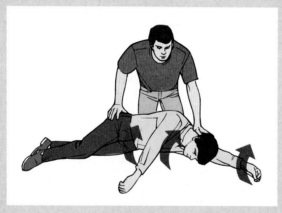

☐ **Roll person onto back (if necessary)**
- Roll person, as one unit, slowly while supporting the head and neck with one hand.

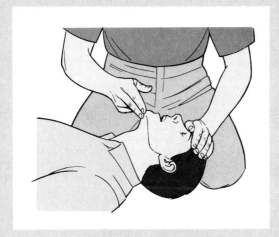

☐ Open airway (use head-tilt/chin-lift)

- Tilt head back and lift chin.

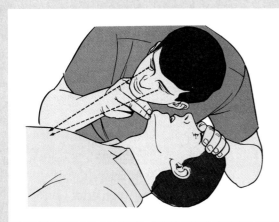

☐ Check for breathing

- Look, listen, and feel for breathing for 3 to 5 seconds.

If person is breathing . . .
- **Put the person in the recovery position.**
- **Keep airway open.**
- **Monitor breathing.**
- **Await arrival of EMS.**

If person is not breathing . . .

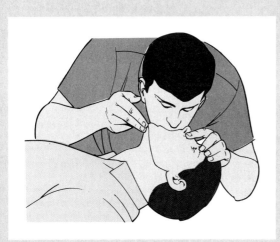

☐ Give 2 slow breaths

- Keep head tilted back.
- Pinch nose shut.
- Seal your lips tightly around person's mouth.
- Give 2 slow breaths.
- Watch chest rise to see that your breaths are going in.

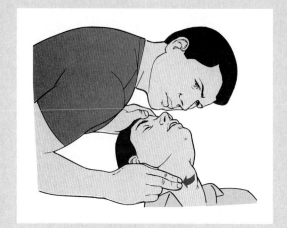

If your breaths go in . . .

☐ **Check for pulse**
- Locate Adam's apple.
- Slide fingers down into groove of neck on side closer to you.
- Feel for pulse for 5 to 10 seconds.

If person does not have a pulse . . .
Begin CPR (see p. 46).
If person has a pulse . . .

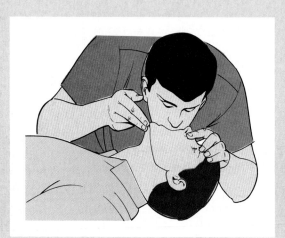

☐ **Continue rescue breathing**
- Maintain open airway with head-tilt/chin-lift.
- Pinch nose shut.
- Give 1 full breath every 5 seconds (about 12 breaths per minute).
- Watch chest rise to see that your breaths are going in.

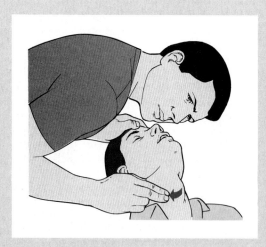

☐ **Recheck pulse and breathing every few minutes**
- Feel for pulse for 5 to 10 seconds.

If person has a pulse and is breathing . . .
- Put the person in the recovery position.
- Keep airway open.
- Monitor breathing.
- Await arrival of EMS.

If person has a pulse but is still not breathing . . .
- Continue rescue breathing until EMS arrives.

If person does not have a pulse and is not breathing . . .
- Begin CPR.
- Await arrival of EMS.

Rescue Breathing for a Child

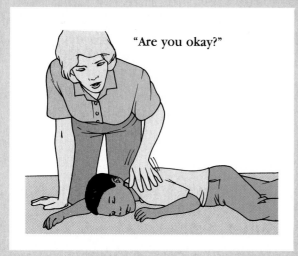

☐ ## Check for consciousness

- Tap or gently shake the child.
- Shout, "Are you OK?"

If the child does not respond . . .

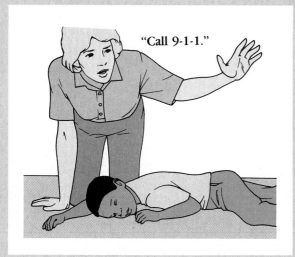

☐ ## Shout for help

- Summon someone who can help and call EMS. If alone, give care for 1 minute, and then call EMS.

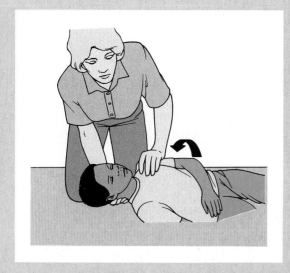

☐ ## Roll the child onto back (if necessary)

- Roll the child, as one unit, by slowly pulling toward you while supporting the head and neck with one hand.

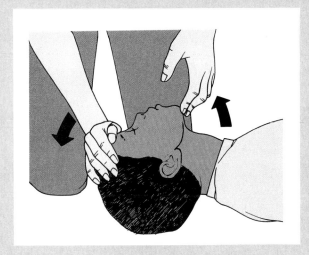

☐ Open airway
- Carefully lift the chin while gently pushing down on the forehead.

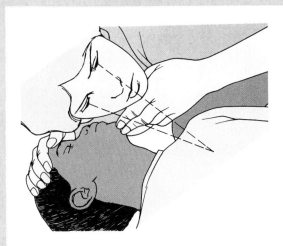

☐ Check for breathing
- Look, listen, and feel for breathing for 3 to 5 seconds.

If the child is breathing. . .
- **Put the child in the recovery position.**
- **Keep airway open.**
- **Monitor breathing.**
- **Phone EMS personnel and await their arrival.**

If the child is not breathing . . .

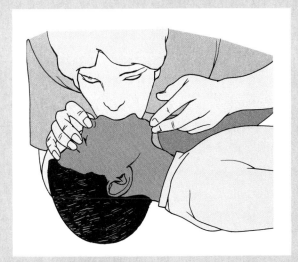

☐ Give 2 slow breaths
- Keep head tilted back.
- Pinch nose shut.
- Seal your lips tightly around the child's mouth.
- Give 2 slow breaths.
- Watch chest rise to see that your breaths are going in.

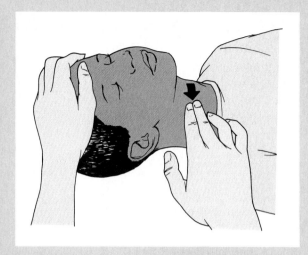

☐ Check for pulse

- Locate Adam's apple.
- Slide fingers down into groove of neck on side closer to you.
- Feel for pulse for 5 to 10 seconds.

If the child does not have a pulse . . .
Begin CPR (see p. 54).
If the child has a pulse . . .

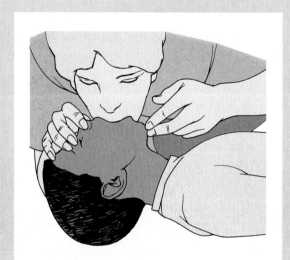

☐ Continue rescue breathing

- Maintain open airway with gentle head-tilt/chin-lift.
- Pinch nose shut.
- Give 1 full breath every 3 seconds.
- Watch chest rise to see that your breaths are going in.
- Continue for 1 minute—about 20 breaths.

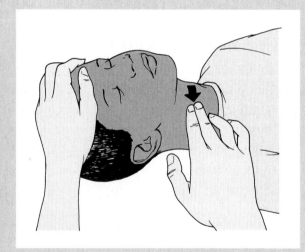

☐ Recheck pulse and breathing every few minutes

- Feel for pulse for 5 to 10 seconds.

If the child has a pulse and is breathing . . .
- Put the child in the recovery position.
- Keep airway open.
- Monitor breathing.
- Await arrival of EMS.

If the child has a pulse but is still not breathing . . .
- Continue rescue breathing until EMS arrives.

If the child does not have a pulse and is not breathing . . .
- Begin CPR.
- Await arrival of EMS.

Rescue Breathing for an Infant

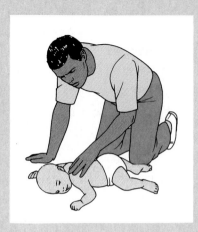

☐ **Check for consciousness**

- Tap or gently shake the infant.
- Call loudly to the infant.

If the infant does not respond . . .

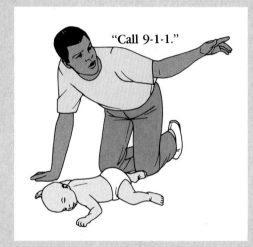

"Call 9-1-1."

☐ **Shout for help**

- Summon someone who can call EMS. If alone, give care for 1 minute, and then call EMS.

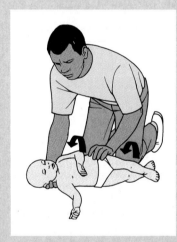

☐ **Roll the infant onto back (if necessary)**

- With one hand on infant's hip and the other on the shoulder and neck supporting the head, roll the infant as one unit.

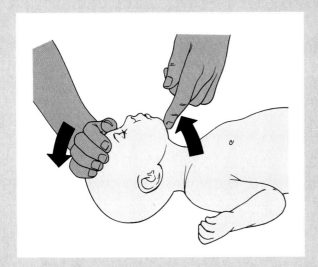

☐ Open airway

- Tilt the infant's head only to a neutral or sniffing position.

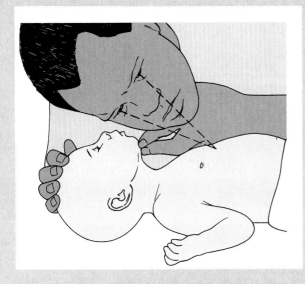

☐ Check for breathing

- Look, listen, and feel for breathing for 3 to 5 seconds.

If the infant is breathing . . .
- **Put the infant in the recovery position.**
- **Keep airway open.**
- **Monitor breathing.**
- **Phone EMS personnel and await their arrival.**

If the infant is not breathing . . .

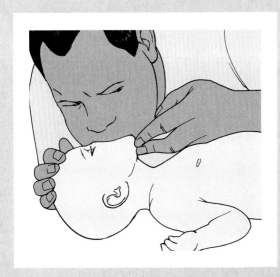

☐ Give 2 slow puffs

- Keep head in neutral or sniffing position.
- Seal your lips tightly over the infant's nose and mouth.
- Give 2 slow puffs, being careful not to force in too much air.
- Watch chest rise to see that your breaths are going in.

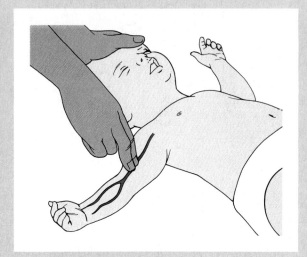

If your breaths go in . . .

☐ Check for pulse

- Check the brachial pulse at the upper part of the arm.
- Feel for pulse for 5 to 10 seconds.

If the infant does not have a pulse . . .
• **Begin CPR (see p. 58).**

If the infant has a pulse . . .

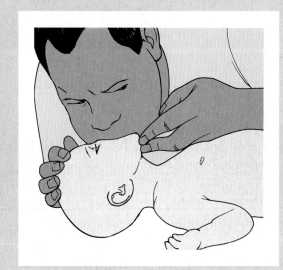

☐ Continue rescue breathing

- Maintain the open airway with head in neutral or sniffing position
- Give 1 puff every 3 seconds.
- Watch chest rise to see that your breaths go in.
- Continue for 1 minute—about 20 breaths.

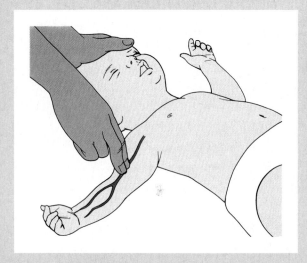

☐ Recheck pulse and breathing every few minutes

- Feel for pulse for 5 to 10 seconds.

If the infant has a pulse and is breathing . . .
• Put in recovery position.
• Keep airway open.
• Monitor breathing.
• Await arrival of EMS.

If the infant has a pulse but is still not breathing . . .
• Continue rescue breathing until EMS arrives.

If the infant does not have a pulse and is not breathing . . .
• Continue CPR until the arrival of EMS.

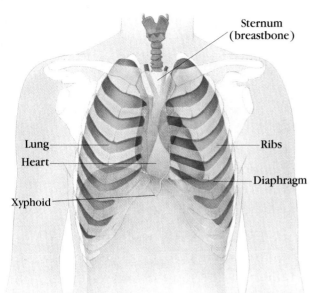

Figure 8 The heart is located in the middle of the chest, behind the lower half of the sternum.

Cardiovascular Emergencies

Cardiovascular emergencies include those illnesses and injuries that affect the circulation, including heart disease, heart attack, stroke, and cardiac arrest. Cardiovascular disease is the leading cause of death for adults in Canada. With over 50,000 Canadians suffering heart attacks each year, it is important to know how to recognize and care for cardiovascular emergencies.

Anatomy and Physiology of Circulation

The heart is a muscular organ that acts like a pump. The ribs and sternum protect it in front and the spine protects it in back (Figure 8). Oxygen-poor blood from the body is brought to the right side of the heart and pumped to the lungs to pick up oxygen. The oxygen-rich blood returns to the left side of the heart and is pumped to all parts of the body. Valves direct the blood through the heart (Figure 9). For the circulatory system to be effective, the respiratory system must also be working so that the blood can pick up oxygen in the lungs.

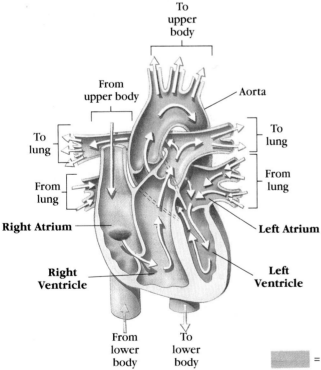

Figure 9 The heart has right and left halves. The right side receives blood from the body and sends it to the lungs. The left side receives blood from the lungs and pumps it out through the body. One-way valves direct the flow of blood through the heart.

= Oxygen-poor blood circulated from the body to the lungs

= Oxygen-rich blood circulated from the lungs to the body

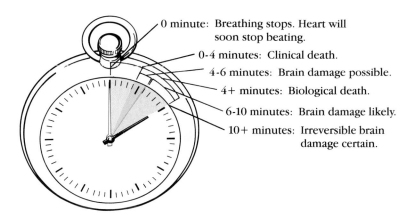

0 minute: Breathing stops. Heart will soon stop beating.

0-4 minutes: Clinical death.

4-6 minutes: Brain damage possible.

4+ minutes: Biological death.

6-10 minutes: Brain damage likely.

10+ minutes: Irreversible brain damage certain.

Figure 10   Time is critical in starting lifesaving measures. Four to six minutes without oxygen generally causes irreversible brain damage.

If the heart stops, the body receives no oxygen. Cells begin to die in 4 to 6 minutes (Figure 10). Some tissues, such as the brain, are very sensitive to oxygen deprivation. If the brain does not receive oxygen within minutes, brain damage or death will result.

Cardiovascular disease, which is disease that affects the heart and blood vessels, develops as cholesterol and other material gradually build up inside the coronary arteries. This condition, called *atherosclerosis*, causes narrowing of the arteries. A clot can completely block a narrowed artery. This process causes both heart attacks and stroke.

Angina

Some people with coronary artery disease sometimes feel intermittent chest pain or pressure, especially with physical activity. This condition is called *angina pectoris*. It develops when the heart needs more oxygen than it is getting. When the coronary arteries have become narrow and the heart needs more oxygen, such as during physical activity, emotional stress, or temperature extremes, heart muscle tissues may not get enough oxygen. This situation causes the pain.

Causes of angina

Any condition that limits the blood to the heart may cause angina. These include coronary artery disease, high blood pressure, anaemia, and certain heart disorders and other diseases.

Heart Attack

Like all tissues, the heart needs continuous oxygen. The coronary arteries bring oxygen to the heart (Figure 11). If heart muscle tissue does not get enough blood, it dies. If too much tissue dies, the heart cannot pump effectively. The sudden blockage of a coronary artery leading to death of heart muscle is called a *heart attack*. A heart attack can cause an irregular heartbeat and prevent blood from circulating effectively.

Causes of heart attack

Heart attack is usually caused by cardiovascular disease. If the coronary arteries bringing blood to the heart muscle are blocked, a heart attack occurs (see Figure 11).

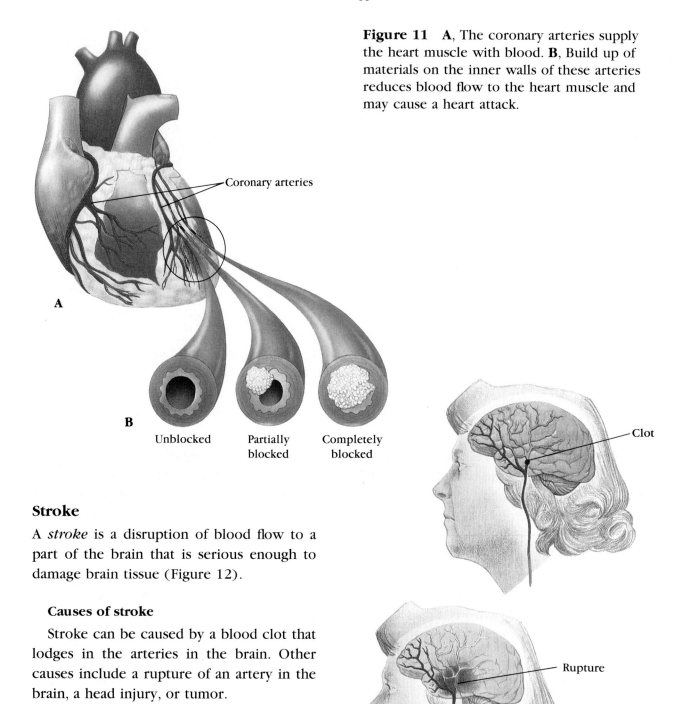

Figure 11 **A**, The coronary arteries supply the heart muscle with blood. **B**, Build up of materials on the inner walls of these arteries reduces blood flow to the heart muscle and may cause a heart attack.

Coronary arteries

A

B

| Unblocked | Partially blocked | Completely blocked |

Clot

Rupture

Stroke

A *stroke* is a disruption of blood flow to a part of the brain that is serious enough to damage brain tissue (Figure 12).

Causes of stroke

Stroke can be caused by a blood clot that lodges in the arteries in the brain. Other causes include a rupture of an artery in the brain, a head injury, or tumor.

Cardiac Arrest

Cardiac arrest occurs when the heart stops beating or beats too irregularly or too weakly to circulate blood effectively. Breathing soon stops. Cardiac arrest is a life-threatening emergency because vital organs can live only a few minutes without oxygen-rich blood.

Figure 12 A stroke can be caused by a blood clot or bleeding from a ruptured artery in the brain.

Causes of cardiac arrest

Cardiovascular disease is the most common cause of cardiac arrest. Drowning, suffocation, and certain drugs can cause breathing to stop, which then causes cardiac arrest. Severe chest injuries or severe blood loss can also cause the heart to beat ineffectively. Electrocution disrupts the heart's own electrical activity and causes the heart to stop.

PREVENTION

Heart Disease

Although a heart attack may seem to strike suddenly, cardiovascular disease develops gradually. A diet high in cholesterol and fats, lack of exercise, high blood pressure, and smoking all contribute to cardiovascular disease, which can begin as early as the teenage years. Prevention of cardiovascular disease and heart attack depends on controlling one's risk factors for developing the disease.

Risk factors for heart disease

Some risk factors for heart disease cannot be changed, such as being a man or having a family history of heart disease.

However many risk factors for heart disease can be controlled. Smoking, a diet high in fats, high blood pressure, obesity, and lack of routine exercise are all risk factors. When one risk factor, such as high blood pressure, is combined with other risk factors, such as obesity or cigarette smoking, the risk of heart attack is greatly increased.

The risk factors for stroke are similar to those for heart disease. You can help prevent stroke by making the same lifestyle changes.

Controlling risk factors

Controlling risk factors means a change in lifestyle to reduce the chances of future disease (Figure 13). The three major controllable risk factors are cigarette smoking, high blood pressure, and intake of fats.

Cigarette smokers have more than twice

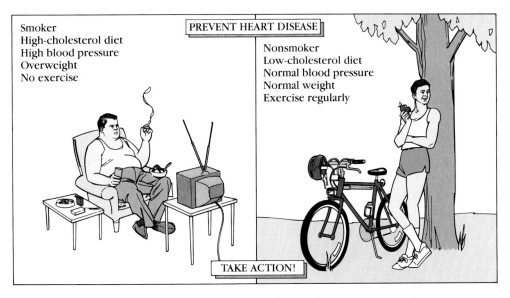

Figure 13   Control risk factors; do not let them control you.

the chance of having a heart attack and two to four times the chance of cardiac arrest than nonsmokers. The earlier a person started using tobacco, the greater the risk. Giving up smoking rapidly reduces the risk of heart disease. After a number of years, the risk becomes the same as if the person never smoked. If you do not smoke, do not start. If you do smoke, quit.

High blood pressure can damage blood vessels in the heart and other organs. You can often control high blood pressure by losing weight, changing your diet, and taking medications when prescribed. Everyone should have regular blood pressure checks.

A diet high in fats and cholesterol increases the risk of heart disease. You should eat only small amounts of foods high in cholesterol, such as egg yolks, organ meats, shrimp, and lobster, and those high in fats, such as beef, lamb, veal, pork, ham, whole milk, and whole milk products. Limiting one's intake is easier than you think. Moderation is the key. Make changes whenever you can by substituting low fat milk or skim milk for whole milk, margarine for butter, trimming visible fat from meats, and broiling or baking rather than frying. Read labels carefully. A "cholesterol free" product may still be high in fat.

Also control your weight and exercise regularly. Excess calories are stored as fat. Obese middle-aged men have nearly three times the risk of a fatal heart attack than nor-

Signs and Symptoms of Cardiovascular Emergencies

Angina

Chest pain that is often described as being tight, heavy, or a pressure and may spread to the neck, jaw, and arms

Pain that usually lasts less than 10 minutes

Pain that is usually relieved by rest

Sometimes associated with difficulty breathing, sweating, nausea, or dizziness

Heart attack

Persistent chest pain or discomfort, usually in the center of the chest or spreading to the shoulder, arm, neck, or jaw.

Difficulty breathing, and faster, slower or irregular pulse.

Skin moist, or sweating profusely; may be pale or bluish in colour in fair-haired casualties.

Nausea and vomiting.

Cardiac arrest

Unconsciousness

Absence of breathing

Absence of pulse

Stroke

Sudden weakness and/or numbness of the face, arm, or leg, usually only on one side of the body

Difficulty talking or understanding speech

Sudden, severe headache

Dizziness or confusion

Unconsciousness

mal-weight middle-aged men. Routine exercise improves muscle tone and helps in weight control. Exercise also improves your chances of surviving a heart attack.

FIRST AID
Cardiovascular Emergencies

First aid for angina

Casualties who know that they have angina usually carry prescribed medication, such as nitroglycerin, with them for the pain. If the casualty asks you, help him or her with the medication. It comes as a small tablet that is placed under the tongue, as a spray used in the mouth, or in patches placed on the chest. Have the casualty sit or lie down. Reducing the heart's demand for oxygen, such as by stopping physical activity, often relieves angina symptoms.

If the person has not been diagnosed by a doctor as having angina, do not ignore this pain because it could be a heart attack. Call EMS immediately and help the casualty rest comfortably.

First aid for a heart attack

The most important thing to do is to recognize any of the heart attack signs and symptoms and take immediate action. A heart attack casualty often denies that the pain or other symptoms are serious. Do not let this change your mind. If you think the person might be having a heart attack, you must act. First, have the casualty stop what he or she is doing and rest comfortably.

If you think the casualty may be having a heart attack or if you are unsure, ask someone to call EMS for help. If you're alone, make the call yourself. Survival following a heart attack often depends on how soon the casualty receives advanced medical care.

Unless EMS services are not readily available, do not try to drive the casualty to the hospital yourself because cardiac arrest can occur at any time. Call the emergency number immediately, before the condition worsens and the heart stops beating.

Keep a calm and reassuring manner when caring for a heart attack casualty. Comfort helps reduce anxiety and eases some of the pain. Watch the casualty closely until EMS arrives. Monitor the casualty's vital signs and watch for changes in appearance or behavior. Since cardiac arrest may occur at any time, be prepared to perform CPR.

First aid for stroke

If there is fluid or vomitus in the casualty's mouth, position him or her in the recovery position with the affected side up. You may have to use a finger sweep to remove some of the material from the mouth. Stay with the casualty until EMS arrives, and monitor his or her ABCs.

First aid for cardiac arrest

A casualty in cardiac arrest needs CPR and emergency medical care immediately. Rescue breathing and chest compressions make the lungs and heart function to some extent. CPR increases the casualty's chances of survival by keeping the brain supplied with oxygen until advanced medical care arrives. Without CPR, the brain dies within 4 to 6 minutes. CPR provides a minimum of the normal blood flow to the brain and heart. Even with CPR, the chance of survival is very slim unless advanced medical care arrives within 10 minutes. Trained emergency personnel can give advanced cardiac life support (ACLS).

CPR for an Adult

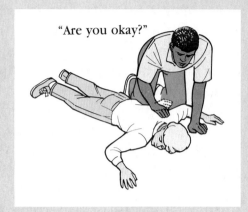

"Are you okay?"

☐ Check for unresponsiveness

- Tap or gently shake person.
- Shout, "Are you OK?"

If person does not respond . . .

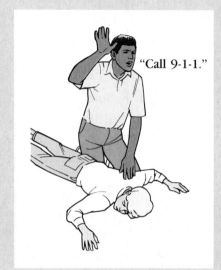

"Call 9-1-1."

☐ Call for help and call EMS

- Summon someone who can help, or call EMS yourself.

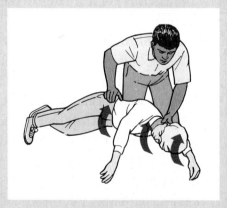

☐ Roll person onto back (if necessary) to check the ABCs.

- Roll person toward you by pulling slowly.

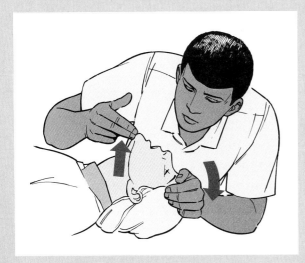

☐ Open airway and check for breathing

- Tilt head back and lift chin.
- Look, listen, and feel for breathing for 3 to 5 seconds.

If person is breathing . . .
- **Put the casualty in the recovery position.**
- **Keep airway open.**
- **Monitor breathing.**

If person is not breathing . . .

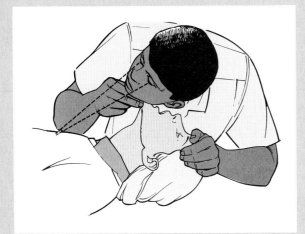

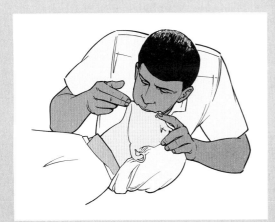

☐ Give 2 slow breaths

- Pinch nose shut and seal your lips tightly around person's mouth.
- Give 2 slow breaths, each lasting 1 1/2 to 2 seconds.
- Watch chest rise to see that your breaths are going in.

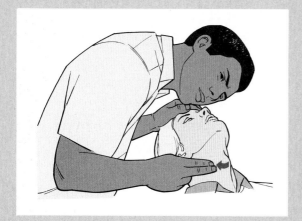

If your breaths go in . . .

☐ Check for pulse

• Feel for pulse for 5 to 10 seconds.

If person has a pulse and is not breathing . . .
• **Continue rescue breathing.**

If person does not have a pulse . . .
• **Begin CPR.**

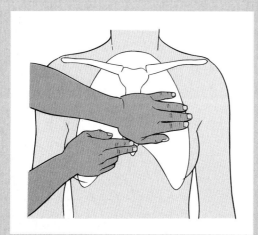

☐ Find hand position

• Locate notch at lower end of sternum, using hand closest to the casualty's feet.
• Place heel of other hand on sternum next to fingers.
• Remove hand from notch and put it on top of other hand.
• Keep fingers off chest.

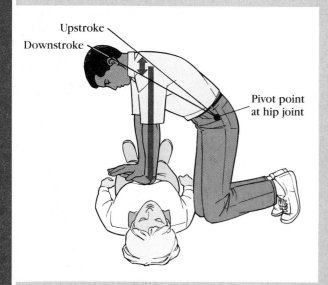

Upstroke
Downstroke

Pivot point at hip joint

☐ Give 15 compressions

• Position shoulders over hands.
• Compress sternum 3.8 to 5 cm (1 1/2 to 2 inches).
• Do 15 compressions in approximately 10 seconds.
• Compress down and up smoothly, keeping hand contact with the chest at all times.

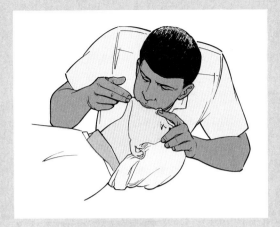

☐ **Give 2 slow breaths**

- Open airway with head-tilt/chin-lift.
- Pinch nose shut and seal your lips tightly around person's mouth.
- Give 2 slow breaths, each lasting 1 1/2 to 2 seconds.
- Watch chest rise to see that your breaths are going in.

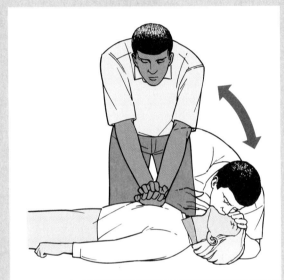

☐ **Repeat compression/ breathing cycles**

- Do 3 more cycles of 15 compressions and 2 breaths.

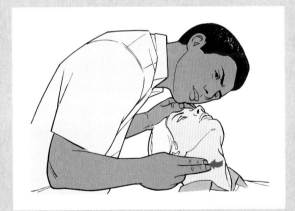

☐ **Recheck pulse and breathing**

- Feel for pulse for about 5 seconds.

If person has a pulse and is breathing . . .
- Put the person in the recovery position.
- Keep airway open.
- Monitor breathing.
- Await arrival of EMS.

If person has a pulse but is still not breathing . . .
- Do rescue breathing until EMS arrives.

If person does not have a pulse and is not breathing . . .
- Continue CPR until EMS arrives.

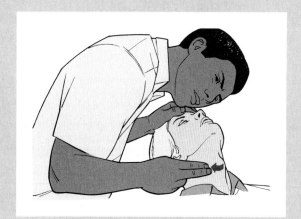

☐ **Recheck pulse and breathing every few minutes.**

Two-Rescuer CPR for an Adult

You are already giving CPR when joined by a second rescuer. The second rescuer first confirms that EMS has been called and then assists you with CPR. As you continue to give chest compressions ask the second rescuer to check the pulse.

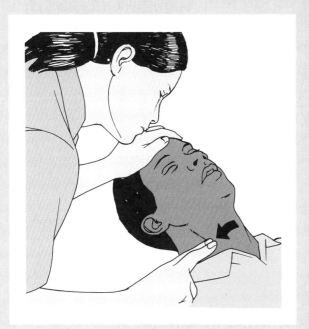

☐ **Second rescuer says, "Stop compressions," and checks pulse for 5 to 10 seconds.**

> **If no pulse, second rescuer gives 1 slow breath.**

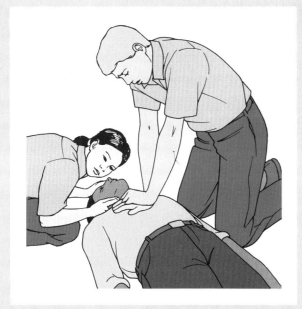

☐ **Give 5 compressions**
  - Position shoulders over hands.
  - Compress sternum 3.8 to 5 cm (1 1/2 to 2 inches).
  - Do 5 compressions. Count aloud so that the second rescuer can join in the cycle.
  - Compress down and up smoothly, keeping hand contact with the chest at all times.
  - Pause after 5 compressions for 1 1/2 to 2 seconds so that second rescuer may give rescue breath.
  - Maintain hand position on sternum, ready to start next cycle of compressions.

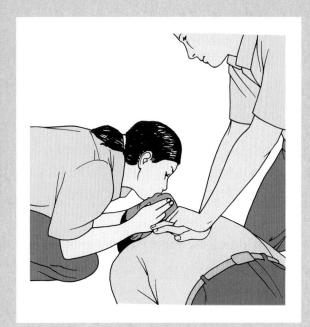

☐ **Second rescuer gives 1 slow breath**

- Second rescuer keeps airway open continuously with head-tilt/chin-lift.
- Second rescuer pinches nose shut and seals lips tightly around person's mouth.
- Second rescuer gives 1 slow breath, lasting 1 1/2 to 2 seconds.
- Second rescuer watches chest rise to see that the breath is going in.

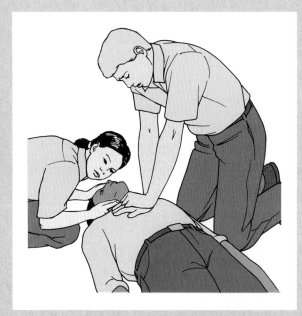

☐ **Continue compression and breathing cycles**

- Give 5 compressions for each breath.

☐ **Second rescuer continually monitors pulse**

- Second rescuer keeps fingers on carotid artery to feel for pulse while keeping the airway open.

If the pulse begins and the casualty starts breathing . . .
- Put the casualty in the recovery position.
- Keep airway open.
- Monitor breathing.
- Await arrival of EMS.

If person has a pulse but is still not breathing . . .
- Do rescue breathing until EMS arrives.

If person does not have a pulse and is not breathing . . .
- Both rescuers continue CPR until EMS arrives.

☐ Continue compression/ breathing cycles

- Continue cycles of 5 compressions, pausing for second rescuer to give 1 breath.

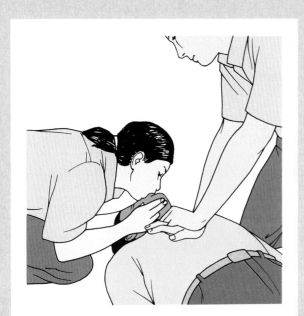

If you become fatigued giving compressions . . .
- Tell second rescuer you want to alternate roles to avoid fatigue.
- Give 5 compressions and pause while second rescuer gives 1 breath.
- Second rescuer finds hand position and begins compressions.
- Monitor carotid pulse continuously and give 1 breath after every 5 compressions.

CPR for a Child

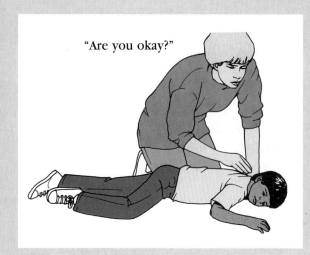

"Are you okay?"

☐ **Check for unresponsiveness**
- Tap or gently shake the child.
- Shout, "Are you OK?"

If the child does not respond . . .

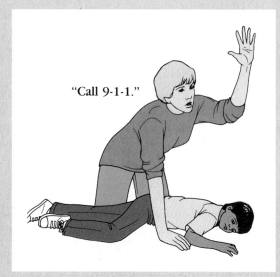

"Call 9-1-1."

☐ **Shout for help**
- Summon someone who can call EMS. If alone, give care for 1 minute, and then call EMS.

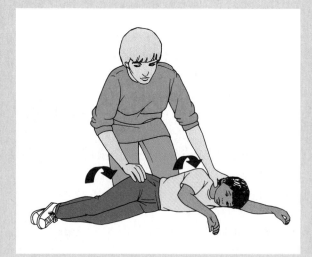

☐ **Roll the child onto back (if necessary)**
- Roll the child toward you by pulling slowly.

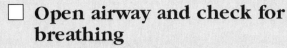
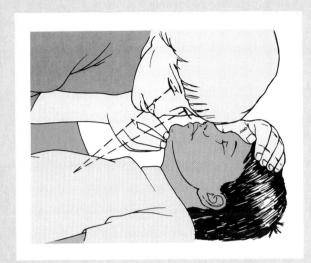

☐ Open airway and check for breathing

- Gently tilt head back and lift chin.
- Look, listen, and feel for breathing for 3 to 5 seconds.

If the child is breathing . . .
- **Put the child in the recovery position.**
- **Keep airway open.**
- **Monitor breathing.**
- **Phone EMS personnel and await their arrival.**

If the child is not breathing . . .

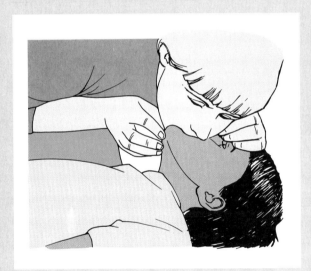

☐ Give 2 slow breaths

- Pinch nose shut and seal your lips tightly around the child's mouth.
- Give 2 slow breaths, each lasting 1 1/2 to 2 seconds, avoiding blowing too forcefully.
- Watch chest rise to see that your breaths are going in.

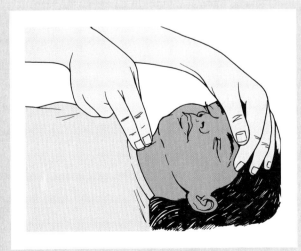

☐ Check for pulse

- Feel for carotid pulse for 5 to 10 seconds.

If the child has a pulse and is not breathing . . .
- **Do rescue breathing.**
- **Phone EMS for help.**

If the child does not have a pulse . . .
- **Begin CPR.**

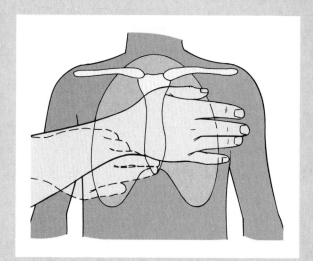

☐ Find hand position

- Locate notch at lower end of sternum.
- Place heel of other hand on sternum next to fingers.
- Use only one hand for compressions.
- Maintain an open airway with the other hand.
- Keep fingers off chest.

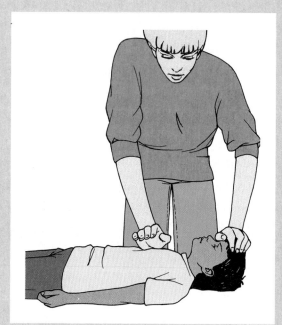

☐ Give 5 compressions

- Position shoulders over hand.
- Compress sternum 2.5 to 3.8 cm (1 to 1 1/2 inches).
- Do 5 compressions in approximately 3 seconds.
- Compress down and up smoothly, keeping hand contact with the chest at all times.

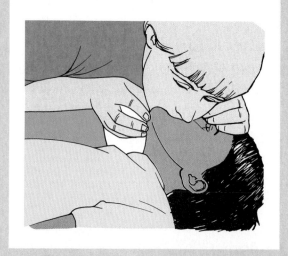

☐ Give 1 slow breath

- Gently open airway with head-tilt/chin-lift.
- Pinch nose shut and seal your lips tightly around child's mouth.
- Give 1 slow breath, lasting 1 1/2 to 2 seconds.
- Watch chest rise to see that your breath is going in.

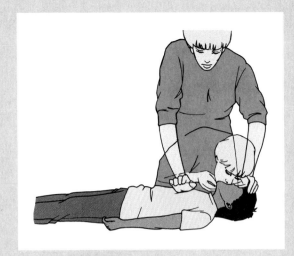

☐ **Repeat compression/ breathing cycles**

- Do 20 cycles of 5 compressions and 1 breath, in total about 60 seconds. If not already done, call EMS.

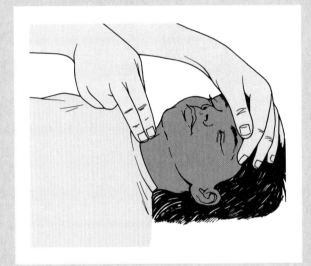

☐ **Recheck pulse and breathing**

- Feel for pulse and check breathing for about 5 seconds.

If the child has a pulse and is breathing . . .
- **Put the child in the recovery position.**
- **Keep airway open.**
- **Monitor breathing.**
- **Await arrival of EMS.**

If the child has a pulse but is still not breathing . . .
- **Do rescue breathing until EMS arrives.**

If the child does not have a pulse and is not breathing . . .
- **Continue CPR until EMS arrives.**

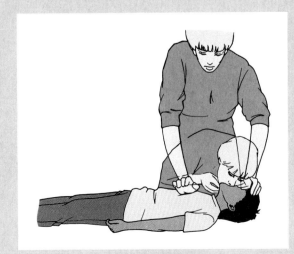

☐ **Continue cycles of 5 compressions and 1 breath, each cycle lasting about 3 seconds**

☐ **Recheck pulse and breathing every few minutes.**

CPR for an Infant

PRACTISE SESSION

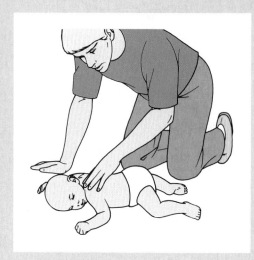

☐ **Check for consciousness**
- Tap or gently shake the infant.
- Call loudly to the infant.

If the infant does not respond . . .

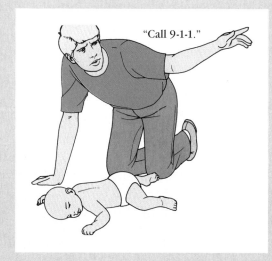

"Call 9-1-1."

☐ **Shout for help**
- Summon someone who can call EMS. If alone, give care for 1 minute, and then call EMS.

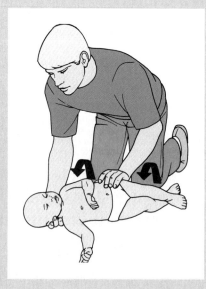

☐ **Roll the infant onto back (if necessary)**
- Roll infant toward you by pulling slowly, being careful to support the head and neck.

56

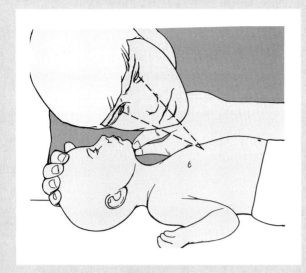

☐ Open airway and check for breathing

- Tilt head to neutral or sniffing position.
- Look, listen, and feel for breathing for 3 to 5 seconds.

If the infant is breathing . . .
- **Put the infant in the recovery position.**
- **Keep airway open.**
- **Monitor breathing.**
- **Phone EMS personnel and await their arrival.**

If the infant is not breathing . . .

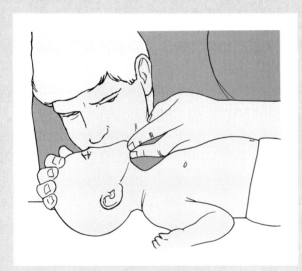

☐ Give 2 slow puffs

- Seal your lips tightly around the infant's nose and mouth.
- Give 2 slow puffs of air, each lasting 1 to 1 1/2 seconds, being careful not to be too forceful.
- Watch chest rise to see that your breaths are going in.

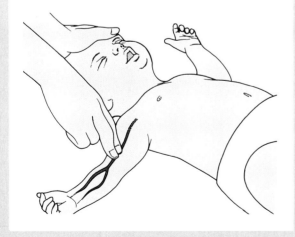

☐ Check for pulse

- Feel for brachial pulse for 5 to 10 seconds.

If the infant has a pulse and is not breathing . . .
- **Do rescue breathing.**
- **Phone EMS for help.**

If the infant does not have a pulse . . .
- **Begin CPR.**

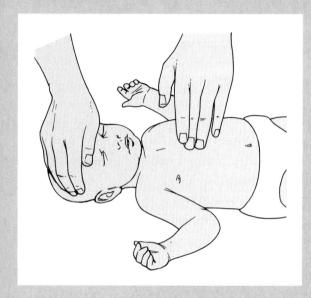

☐ Find correct finger position

- Place middle three fingers with index finger on the line between the nipples.
- Lift index finger, so that middle and ring fingers are on sternum below the nipple line.

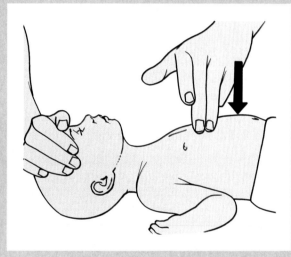

☐ Give 5 compressions

- Compress sternum 1.2 to 2.5 cm (1/2 to 1 inch).
- Do 5 compressions in approximately 3 seconds.
- Compress down and up smoothly, keeping fingers in contact with the chest at all times.

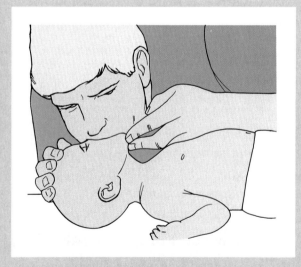

☐ Give 1 slow puff

- Open airway by tilting head to neutral or sniffing position.
- Seal your lips tightly around the infant's nose and mouth.
- Give 1 slow puff of air.
- Watch chest rise to see that your breath is going in.

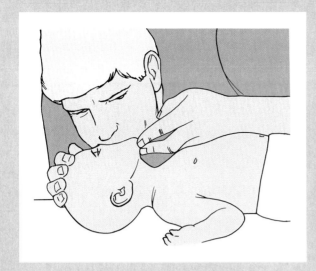

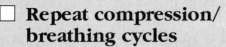

☐ Repeat compression/ breathing cycles

- Do 20 cycles of 5 compressions and 1 breath, in total about 60 seconds. If not already done, call EMS.

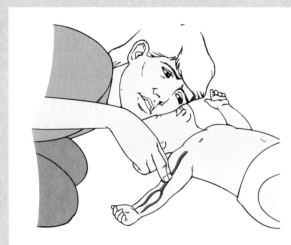

☐ Recheck breathing and pulse (for about 5 seconds)

If the infant is breathing and has a pulse . . .
- **Put infant in the recovery position.**
- **Keep airway open.**
- **Monitor breathing.**
- **Await arrival of EMS.**

If the infant is not breathing and has no pulse . . .
- **Continue CPR until EMS arrives.**

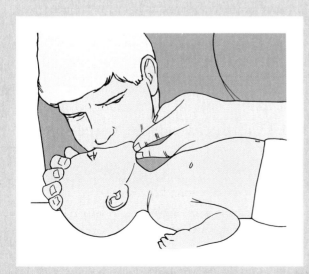

☐ Continue cycles of 5 compressions and 1 breath, each cycle lasting 3 seconds.

☐ Recheck breathing every few minutes.

Appendix A

Common Questions about Cardiovascular Health and First Aid

Cardiovascular Health

Q. What is a TIA?

A. A transient ischemic attack (TIA) is a temporary episode, often called a little stroke, that is caused by a reduction in the blood flow to a part of the brain. Unlike a stroke, it is temporary and lasts anywhere from 10 minutes to 24 hours. A TIA is an early warning sign of stroke. Casualties should seek medical attention.

Q. How do I know if I have high blood pressure?

A. Most of the time a person with high blood pressure (hypertension) feels healthy and has no symptoms. Only by getting a blood pressure check can you know if you have high blood pressure. High blood pressure is a risk factor for cardiovascular disease and thus needs to be controlled through diet, exercise, and, sometimes, medication. All of us should have our blood pressure checked regularly.

Q. What is the silent killer?

A. The silent killer, high blood pressure, is called this because the person usually feels no symptoms. However, high blood pressure can lead to heart attack, stroke, or other cardiovascular disease. (See the preceding question.)

Special Considerations for First Aid for Choking

Q. Should you try to give abdominal thrusts to a person who is pregnant or very large?

A. Give chest thrusts to a noticeably pregnant woman, an unconscious casualty, or any larger adult to whom you cannot deliver abdominal thrusts effectively. Kneel facing the casualty. Place the heel of one hand on the center of the casualty's breastbone and

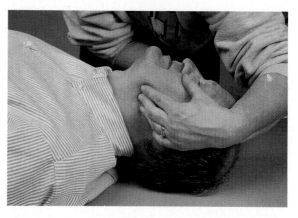

Figure 14 Use the jaw thrust method for opening the airway if the casualty has a neck or back injury or if the head-tilt/chin-lift method does not succeed.

your other hand on top of it. Give 5 quick thrusts. Each thrust should compress the chest 3.5 to 5 cm (1.5 to 2 inches). After giving 5 chest thrusts, do a finger sweep, open the airway, and give 2 full breaths as you normally would for an unconscious choking adult. Repeat the sequence until the obstruction is dislodged, you can breathe into the casualty, or EMS arrives and takes over.

Q. How should one open the airway of a casualty who may have a head, neck, or back injury?

A. Suspect head, neck, or back injuries in casualties who have experienced a violent force, such as in a motor vehicle crash, a fall, or a diving or sports injury. In such cases minimize movement of the head and neck when opening the airway. Use the jaw thrust method instead of the head-tilt/chin-lift (Figure 14).

Special Considerations for Rescue Breathing

Q. Is it possible to blow air into the stomach when giving rescue breathing?

A. Air normally goes into the casualty's lungs, but in some cases it may enter the stomach instead. Be careful of three things. (1) Do not overinflate the lungs; stop the breath when the chest has risen. (2) If the casualty's head is not tilted back far enough, the airway will not open completely and the chest may only rise slightly, leading you to breathe more forcefully, causing air to enter the stomach. (3) If you give breaths too quickly, increased pressure in the airway causes air to enter the stomach; long, slow breaths minimize pressure in the air passages. Air in the stomach can make the casualty vomit. When an unconscious person vomits, stomach contents may get into the lungs, a situation that hampers rescue breathing and can be fatal.

Q. Is it true that casualties often vomit during rescue breathing or CPR?

A. Even without air in the stomach, casualties often vomit when given rescue breathing. If this happens, turn the casualty's head and body together as a unit onto one side. This helps prevent vomit from entering the lungs. Quickly wipe the casualty's mouth clean, reposition the casualty on his or her back, and continue with rescue breathing.

Q. Can you ever give rescue breathing through the nose?

A. Sometimes you cannot seal your mouth well over the casualty's mouth to give rescue breathing. The person's jaw or mouth may be injured or shut too tightly to open, or your mouth may be too small to cover the casualty's. If so, hold the mouth closed and give rescue breathing through the casualty's nose.

Q. How do you give rescue breathing to a casualty with a stoma?

A. People who have had an operation that removed part of their windpipe breathe through an opening in the front of the neck called a *stoma*. Air passes directly into the windpipe through the stoma instead of through the mouth and nose. Therefore you give rescue breathing through the stoma.

Q. Should you remove a casualty's dentures before giving rescue breathing?

A. If you know or see that the casualty is wearing dentures, do not automatically remove them. Dentures help rescue breathing by supporting the casualty's mouth and cheeks during mouth-to-mouth breathing. If the dentures are loose, the head-tilt/chin-lift may help keep them in place. Remove the dentures *only* if they become so loose that they block the airway or make it difficult for you to give breaths.

Special Considerations for CPR

Q. When is it okay to stop giving CPR?

A. Once you begin CPR, stop only if:

- Your personal safety is threatened.
- The casualty's heart starts to beat on its own.
- Another trained rescuer arrives on the scene and takes over.
- You are too exhausted to continue.

Appendix B

Prevention of Injuries to Children

Use this checklist to spot dangers in your home. When you read each question, circle either the "Yes" box or the "No" box. Each "No" shows a possible danger for you and your family. Work with your family to remove dangers and make your home safer.

General Safety Precautions Inside the Home

Yes   No

☐ ☐ Are stairways kept clear and uncluttered?

☐ ☐ Are stairs and hallways well lit?

☐ ☐ Are safety gates installed at tops and bottoms of stairways?

☐ ☐ Are guards installed around fireplaces, radiators or hot pipes, and wood-burning stoves?

☐ ☐ Are sharp edges of furniture cushioned with corner guards or other material?

☐ ☐ Are unused electric outlets covered with tape or safety covers?

☐ ☐ Are curtain cords and shade pulls kept out of child's reach?

☐ ☐ Are windows secured with window locks?

☐ ☐ Are plastic bags kept out of child's reach?

☐ ☐ Are fire extinguishers installed where they are most likely to be needed?

☐ ☐ Are smoke detectors in working order?

☐ ☐ Do you have an emergency plan to use in case of fire? Does your family practice this plan?

☐ ☐ Is the water set at a safe temperature. (A setting of 120° F or less prevents scalding from tap water in sinks and tubs. Let the water run for three minutes before testing it.)

☐ ☐ If you have a gun, is it locked in a place where your child cannot get it?

☐ ☐ Are all purses, handbags, brief cases, and so on, including those of visitors, kept out of child's reach?

☐ ☐ Are all poisonous plants kept out of child's reach?

☐ ☐ Is a list of emergency phone numbers posted near a telephone?

☐ ☐ Is a list of instructions posted near a telephone for use by children and/or babysitters?

☐ ☐ Do you constantly check the environment and all toys for small objects that the infant or young child may put in the mouth?

☐ ☐ Do you keep young children away from balloons, which can burst into small pieces that can be easily inhaled or ingested?

☐ ☐ Have you removed any items with cords, belts, or other parts that could be wrapped around the child's neck?

Kitchen

Yes   No

☐ ☐ Do you cook on back stove burners when possible and turn pot handles toward the back of the stove?

☐ ☐ Are hot dishes kept away from the edges of tables and counters?

☐ ☐ Are hot liquids and foods kept out of child's reach?

☐ ☐ Are knives and other sharp items kept out of child's reach?

❏ ❏ Is the highchair placed away from stove and other hot appliances?

❏ ❏ Are matches and lighters kept out of child's reach?

❏ ❏ Are all appliance cords kept out of child's reach?

❏ ❏ Are cabinets equipped with safety latches?

❏ ❏ Are cabinet doors kept closed when not in use?

❏ ❏ Are cleaning products kept out of child's reach?

❏ ❏ Do you test the temperature of heated food before feeding the child?

❏ ❏ Do you feed children only when they are seated in a high chair or a secure seat?

❏ ❏ Do you prevent young children from moving about with food in their hands or mouth?

❏ ❏ Do you feed an infant or young child only appropriate soft foods in small pieces?

❏ ❏ Do you constantly watch the child when eating?

Bathroom

Yes **No**

❏ ❏ Are the toilet seat and lid kept down when the toilet is not in use?

❏ ❏ Are cabinets equipped with safety latches and kept closed?

❏ ❏ Are all medicines in child-resistant containers and stored in a locked medicine cabinet?

❏ ❏ Are shampoos and cosmetics stored out of child's reach?

❏ ❏ Are razors, razor blades, and other sharp objects kept out of child's reach?

❏ ❏ Are hair dryers and other appliances stored away from sink, tub, and toilet?

❏ ❏ Does the bottom of tub or shower have rubber stickers or a rubber mat to prevent slipping?

❏ ❏ Is the child always watched by an adult while in the tub?

Child's Room

Yes **No**

❏ ❏ Is child's bed or crib placed away from radiators and other hot surfaces?

❏ ❏ Are crib slats no more than 2⅜ inches apart?

❏ ❏ Does the mattress fit the sides of the crib snugly?

❏ ❏ Is paint or finish on furniture and toys nontoxic?

❏ ❏ Are electric cords kept out of child's reach?

❏ ❏ Is the child's clothing, especially sleepwear, flame resistant?

❏ ❏ Does the toy box have a secure lid and safeclosing hinges?

❏ ❏ Are the toys in good repair?

❏ ❏ Are toys appropriate for child's age?

Parent's Bedroom

Yes **No**

❏ ❏ Are space heaters kept away from curtains and flammable materials?

❏ ❏ Are cosmetics, perfumes, and breakable items stored out of child's reach?

❏ ❏ Are small objects, such as jewelry, buttons, and safety pins, kept out of child's reach?

Storage Area

Yes   No

☐   ☐   Are pesticides, detergents, and other household chemicals kept out of child's reach?

☐   ☐   Are tools kept out of child's reach?

☐   ☐   Have you removed the doors from old refrigerators and similar containers where a child could be trapped?

Outside the Home/Play Area

Yes   No

☐   ☐   Is trash kept in tightly covered containers?

☐   ☐   Are walkways, stairs, and railings in good repair?

☐   ☐   Are walkways and stairs free of toys, tools, and other objects?

☐   ☐   Are sandboxes and wading pools covered when not in use?

☐   ☐   Are swimming pools nearby enclosed with a fence that your child cannot easily climb over?

☐   ☐   Is playground equipment safe? Is it assembled according to the manufacturer's instructions and anchored over a level, soft surface such as sand or wood chips?

☐   ☐   Do you always take steps to prevent drowning by using approved life jackets around water and following safe water recreation practices?

Child Safety IQ

☐ Do you buckle your child into an approved automobile safety seat even when making short trips?

☐ Do you teach your child safety by behaving safely in your own everyday activities?

☐ Do you supervise your child whenever he or she is around water and maintain fences and gates that act as barriers to water?

☐ Have you checked your home for potential fire hazards? Are smoke detectors installed and working?

☐ Are all poisonous substances — cleaning supplies, medicines, plants, etc.— kept out of a child's reach?

☐ Are foods and small items that can choke a child kept out of reach?

☐ Have you inspected your home, day-care center, school, babysitter's home, or wherever your child spends time for potential safety and health hazards?

☐ Do you keep guns and ammunition stored separately and locked up?